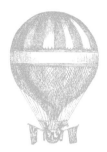

OPTIMISTS LIVE LONGER
INSPIRATIONAL QUOTES

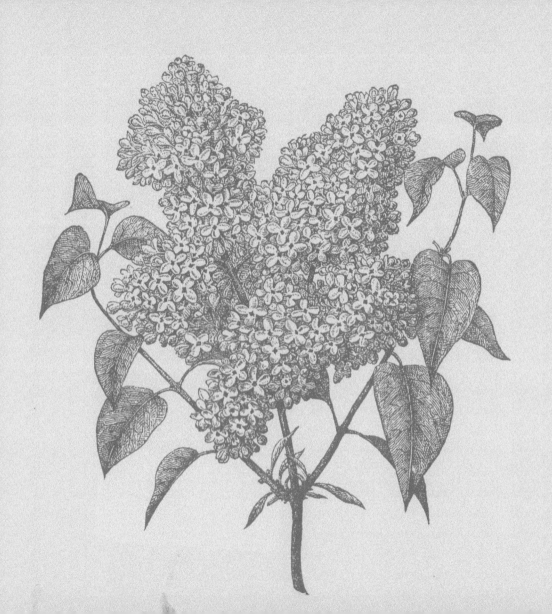

OPTIMISTS LIVE LONGER

INSPIRATIONAL QUOTES

WORDS TO INSPIRE POSITIVE THINKING

 ALEXA BRAND, MS, LMFT

ROCKRIDGE
PRESS

Interior and Cover Designer: Patricia Fabricant
Art Producer: Alyssa Williams
Production Editor: Holland Baker
Production Manager: Martin Worthington
Illustrations © Brigantine Designs/Creative Market and © Beehouse Studio/Creative Market

Paperback ISBN: 978-1-63807-977-4
eBook ISBN: 978-1-63807-649-0
R0

To you accepting yourself unconditionally

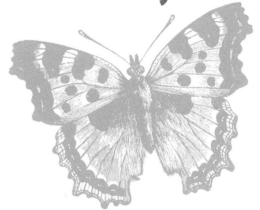

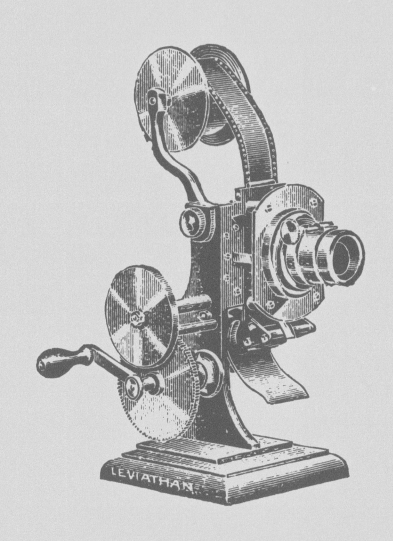

INTRODUCTION

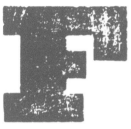or most of my life, I battled with my inner critic. I always needed to do better and be better. But whatever I tried, it was never enough—I was never enough. I resisted uncomfortable emotions and thought I needed to be harder on myself to achieve happiness and success. Sound familiar? Little did I realize that my resistance and self-critical approach was only making things worse, fueling anxiety, depression, disordered eating, and toxic relationships. It wasn't until I found the power of positive thinking on my own journey of healing that I began to feel content in my life. That's not to say I don't still have challenging thoughts or encounter rough patches. But now I have the tools to move through these moments with more understanding and grace. I am able to heal via

the self-compassion, radical acceptance, and gratitude I've fostered with positive thinking. That's why I wrote this book: I want to empower you with the same tools that empowered me. I want to help you use positive thinking to step into your authentic self, move through challenging times, and find your aligned path.

Every person I have worked with as a therapist has struggled with their inner critic and tends to grapple with finding happiness in the present. The world is always telling you that you are insufficient and that you need more (stuff, money, friends, etc.) to be happy. You even may have internalized shame messages received at a young age. Those who are marginalized in society have had additional layers of negative messages sent their way.

If any of this resonates with you, know you are not alone. Thankfully, there is help.

Boosting your mind and heart with positivity is key! Even the smallest moments of positivity make a significant impact on your life. Challenging your negative thoughts, affirming your resilience, and showing up for yourself nonjudgmentally are just a few examples of how to bring positivity into your life. This is what the quotes, information, and tools in this book are here to help you foster. You do not have to read this book in any particular order; simply drop into the pages that call out to you. If you feel discouraged, don't give up. Feeling this way does not indicate failure. It's human to feel disappointed every once in a while. Take a moment to review the Power Positivity sections at these times. Let this book provide you with inspiration and guidance to continue on your positive thinking journey. Above all, remember that you've got this!

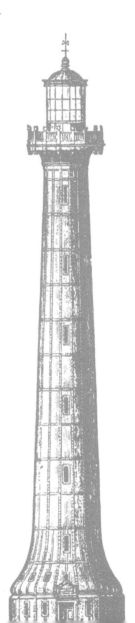

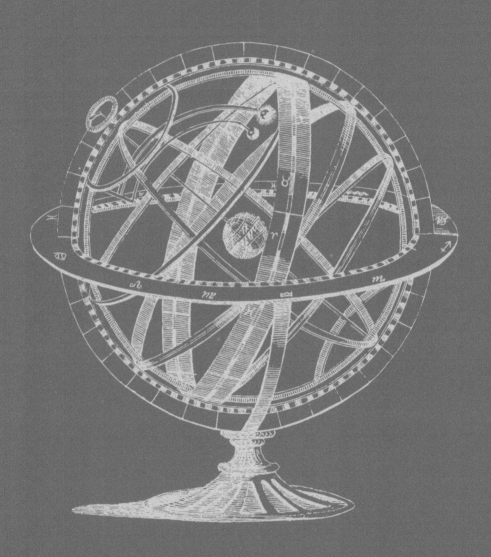

IF ONE ADVANCES CONFIDENTLY
IN THE DIRECTION OF HIS DREAMS,
AND ENDEAVORS TO LIVE THE
LIFE WHICH HE HAS IMAGINED,
HE WILL MEET WITH A SUCCESS
UNEXPECTED IN COMMON HOURS.

—HENRY DAVID THOREAU,
TRANSCENDENTALIST PHILOSOPHER

Believe you can and you're halfway there.

—THEODORE ROOSEVELT,
26TH PRESIDENT OF THE UNITED STATES

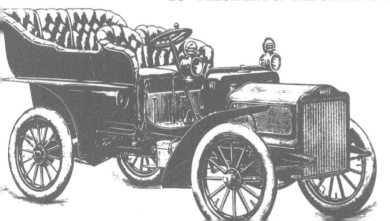

EVERYTHING CAN BE TAKEN FROM A MAN BUT ONE THING: THE LAST OF THE HUMAN FREEDOMS—TO CHOOSE ONE'S ATTITUDE IN ANY GIVEN SET OF CIRCUMSTANCES, TO CHOOSE ONE'S OWN WAY.

—VIKTOR FRANKL,
PSYCHIATRIST, PHILOSOPHER, AND HOLOCAUST SURVIVOR

WITHOUT COURAGE, WE CANNOT PRACTICE ANY OTHER VIRTUE WITH CONSISTENCY. WE CAN'T BE KIND, TRUE, MERCIFUL, GENEROUS, OR HONEST.

—MAYA ANGELOU, AUTHOR
AND CIVIL RIGHTS ACTIVIST

LET YOURSELF BECOME THAT SPACE THAT WELCOMES ANY EXPERIENCE WITHOUT JUDGEMENT.

—TSOKNYI RINPOCHE, BUDDHIST TEACHER

POWER POSITIVITY:
PRACTICE GRATITUDE

Each night, before you drift off to sleep, reflect on your day and write down one thing for which you are grateful. A study published in *Psychotherapy Research* found that people who wrote gratitude letters experienced significantly better mental health than those who didn't. Gratitude goes a step beyond being thankful. Expressing gratitude is truly appreciating certain aspects of yourself and others, as well as the situations and circumstances of your life. It's easy to get stuck in a negative thinking cycle that distracts you from appreciating all that is going well or even just going okay. However, getting in the habit of practicing gratitude can help! Even more exciting, *Harvard Health Publishing* found that most research supports the idea that gratitude is connected to your overall well-being.

WHEN YOU HAVE A DREAM, YOU'VE GOT TO GRAB IT AND NEVER LET IT GO.

—CAROL BURNETT, COMEDIAN AND ACTOR

THE MOST COMMON WAY PEOPLE GIVE UP THEIR POWER IS BY THINKING THEY DON'T HAVE ANY.

—ALICE WALKER, PULITZER PRIZE—WINNING AUTHOR

DON'T BE SATISFIED WITH STORIES, HOW THINGS HAVE GONE WITH OTHERS. UNFOLD YOUR OWN MYTH.

—RUMI, 13TH CENTURY POET AND SCHOLAR

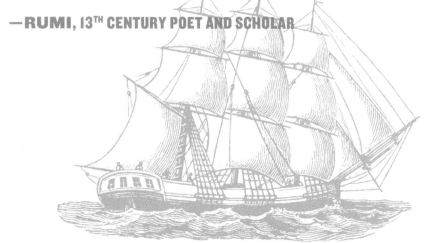

PRACTICE SHARING THE
FULLNESS OF YOUR
BEING, YOUR BEST SELF,
YOUR ENTHUSIASM,
YOUR VITALITY, YOUR
SPIRIT, YOUR TRUST,
YOUR OPENNESS, ABOVE
ALL, YOUR PRESENCE.

—JON KABAT-ZINN,
CREATOR OF MINDFULNESS-BASED STRESS REDUCTION

NOW AND THEN IT'S GOOD TO PAUSE IN OUR PURSUIT OF HAPPINESS AND JUST BE HAPPY.

—GUILLAUME APOLLINAIRE,
AUTHOR AND ART CRITIC

POWER POSITIVITY:
LEARN TO LAUGH AT YOURSELF

Did you know that humor is good for your healing and physical health? When you laugh, you increase your oxygen intake, which pumps up the feel-good hormones in your brain. This relieves stress and increases muscle relaxation. In the long term, it can improve your immune system and heart health, aid your memory and sleep, relieve physical pain, and create positive shifts in your mindset. So don't always take yourself too seriously. When you laugh at yourself, you allow yourself to let go of your inner critic while making room for compassion and positivity. Laughter is contagious, so flex your laughter muscles by seeking out comedy and spending time with people who are lighthearted. By honing your ability to laugh easily and often, you can reap the many healing benefits a good chuckle provides.

IN THREE WORDS I CAN SUM UP EVERYTHING I'VE LEARNED ABOUT LIFE: IT GOES ON.

—ROBERT FROST,
PULITZER PRIZE–WINNING POET

He who has a "why" to live for can bear almost any "how."

—FRIEDRICH NIETZSCHE, PHILOSOPHER

YOU CANNOT LOVE WHAT YOU CANNOT SEE AFRESH. YOU CANNOT LOVE WHAT YOU ARE NOT CONSTANTLY DISCOVERING ANEW.

—ANTHONY DE MELLO,
JESUIT PRIEST AND PSYCHOTHERAPIST

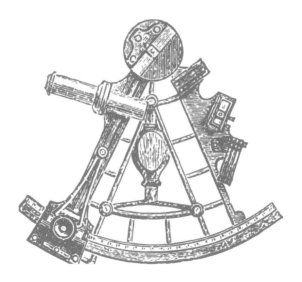

IT IS NOT I WHO CREATE MYSELF, RATHER I HAPPEN TO MYSELF.

—CARL JUNG,
PSYCHIATRIST, PSYCHOANALYST, AND
FOUNDER OF ANALYTICAL PSYCHOLOGY

NO MATTER WHAT YOU'RE GOING THROUGH, THERE'S A LIGHT AT THE END OF THE TUNNEL.

—DEMI LOVATO,
GRAMMY AWARD–WINNING POP SINGER

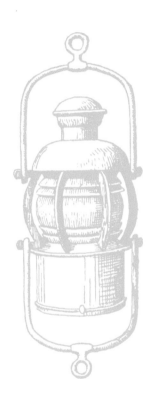

POWER POSITIVITY:
CHALLENGE YOUR THOUGHTS

Positive thinking is the ability to be aware of your thoughts and challenge toxic ways of thinking. Toxic thoughts are those that can keep you stuck in harmful patterns or lead you to more destructive ones. Combining mindfulness with cognitive behavioral therapy (CBT) can help you identify and confront negative patterns of thinking. Ask yourself:

❋ Is this thought actually true? Do I have proof that this thought is true? Is there evidence that this thought is wrong?

❋ Is this thought keeping me stuck in a toxic pattern? Or is this thought allowing me to grow? What evidence do I have of this?

❋ Is this thought self-critical? Or is this thought showing myself kindness and understanding?

❋ Am I engaging in all-or-nothing (black-or-white) thinking? Or am I seeing the gray areas?

❋ What would a trusted loved one say about this thought?

❋ Is there another way to look at this problem? Is there a perspective I'm not seeing at the moment?

Nothing is impossible. The word itself says "I'm possible!"

—AUDREY HEPBURN,
ACADEMY AWARD–WINNING ACTOR AND
GOODWILL AMBASSADOR OF UNICEF

THE MIND DOES NOT
REQUIRE FILLING LIKE A
BOTTLE, BUT RATHER,
LIKE WOOD, IT ONLY
REQUIRES KINDLING.

—PLUTARCH, PHILOSOPHER

LET'S BEGIN BY TAKING A SMALLISH NAP OR TWO.

—A. A. MILNE, AUTHOR

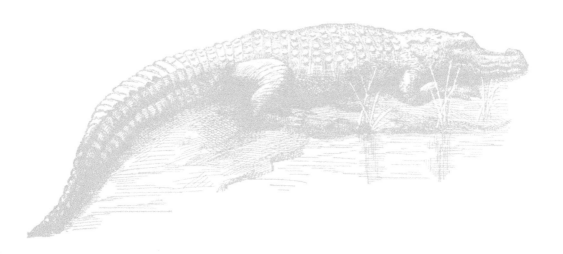

IN A SOCIETY THAT PROFITS FROM YOUR SELF-DOUBT, LIKING YOURSELF IS A REBELLIOUS ACT.

—CAROLINE CALDWELL, ARTIST AND WRITER

Do your thing and don't care if they like it.

—TINA FEY, ACTOR AND COMEDIAN

POWER POSITIVITY: PRIORITIZE REST

Are you always on the move? Most of my clients rarely take time for themselves, which leads to an unfortunate consequence: burnout. Burnout is the negative mental impact that occurs when you're so busy you don't leave any space for downtime. Burnout shows up as emotional exhaustion (anxiety, depression, agitation, numbness, detachment that leads to isolation, loss of pleasure, apathy, and hopelessness), cognitive exhaustion (impaired concentration, attention, and memory), and/or physical exhaustion (chronic fatigue, insomnia, and a weakened immune system).

How do you avoid burnout? Rest! Rest both prevents and cures burnout. It's common to equate rest with being lazy in our productivity-focused culture, but that's simply not true. In fact, Dr. Alex Soojung-Kim Pang, an expert on the topic, has found in his research that rest actually *increases* creativity and productivity. Here are three easy ways to integrate more rest into your life:

- ❋ Take a five-minute rest period for every hour of work you do.
- ❋ Go to bed 15 minutes earlier than usual.
- ❋ Plan a relaxing activity you do by yourself.

Remember, rest is restorative!

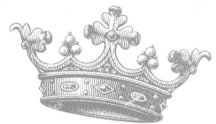

I am a queen because I know how to govern myself.

—LAILAH GIFTY AKITA,
AUTHOR AND FOUNDER OF SMART YOUTH
VOLUNTEERS FOUNDATION

YOU ARE NEVER TOO OLD TO SET ANOTHER GOAL OR TO DREAM A NEW DREAM.

—LES BROWN, MOTIVATIONAL SPEAKER

THE OAK FOUGHT THE WIND AND WAS BROKEN, THE WILLOW BENT WHEN IT MUST AND SURVIVED.

—ROBERT JORDAN, AUTHOR

SINCE
MY HOUSE
BURNED
DOWN I
NOW HAVE
A BETTER
VIEW OF THE
RISING MOON.

—MIZUTA MASAHIDE,
17TH CENTURY POET AND SAMURAI

DO NOT JUDGE ME BY MY SUCCESSES, JUDGE ME BY HOW MANY TIMES I FELL DOWN AND GOT BACK UP AGAIN.

—NELSON MANDELA,
ANTI-APARTHEID REVOLUTIONARY,
POLITICAL LEADER, AND PHILANTHROPIST

POWER POSITIVITY:
GET IN THE FLOW

Have you ever been so engrossed in a creative activity that you completely lost track of time or forgot to be self-conscious? Creative outlets are super powerful and can positively impact your mental health! Mihaly Csikszentmihalyi, one of the founders of positive psychology, discovered that entering a state of flow brings deep pleasure. Finding flow is all about challenging yourself in your creative area of passion. However, you don't want to make the challenge too difficult; it's all about finding the middle ground. Create time and space to focus on your creative outlet and set a realistic goal. For example, set aside time on a Sunday afternoon to paint (or code, or whatever else floats your boat!) and challenge yourself to practice one new manageable technique. When you are done, reflect on your experience. Were you able to achieve a flow? How did it impact your mood? If you struggle to find your flow, that's okay! Try out a different skill next time. Sometimes it takes finding the specific practice that works best for you.

ONLY THOSE WHO DARE TO FAIL GREATLY CAN EVER ACHIEVE GREATLY.

—ROBERT F. KENNEDY,
LAWYER, POLITICIAN, AND 64TH ATTORNEY
GENERAL OF THE UNITED STATES

ALTHOUGH THE WORLD IS FULL OF SUFFERING, IT IS FULL ALSO OF THE OVERCOMING OF IT. MY OPTIMISM, THEN, DOES NOT REST ON THE ABSENCE OF EVIL, BUT ON A GLAD BELIEF IN THE PREPONDERANCE OF GOOD AND A WILLING EFFORT ALWAYS TO COOPERATE WITH THE GOOD, THAT IT MAY PREVAIL.

—HELEN KELLER,
AUTHOR, DISABILITY RIGHTS ADVOCATE,
AND POLITICAL ACTIVIST

WE NEED THE COURAGE TO LEARN FROM OUR PAST AND NOT LIVE IN IT.

—SHARON SALZBERG,
AUTHOR AND BUDDHIST TEACHER

TO "LIVE TRUE" WE NEED TO
AWAKEN SELF-COMPASSION
AND LOVE OURSELVES INTO
HEALING. AND WE NEED TO
ATTUNE TO OTHERS WITH AN
ACTIVE CARING, AND INCLUDE
ALL BEINGS IN OUR HEART.

—TARA BRACH,
PSYCHOLOGIST AND MEDITATION TEACHER

Time you enjoy wasting is not wasted time.

—MARTHE TROLY-CURTIN, AUTHOR

POWER POSITIVITY: EMBRACE AFFIRMATIONS

Positive affirmations are simple statements of self-talk that help boost your mood! Research by Cohen and Sherman shows that practicing affirmations decreases stress and negative ruminations and increases self-worth. Therefore, positive affirmations are a powerful tool to help you in your positive thinking journey. Here are 10 examples of affirmations you can repeat to yourself to promote positivity:

1. Today, I choose to think positively.
2. I believe in myself.
3. I can overcome any challenges that arise.
4. I am grateful for all that I have.
5. Each day, I am learning and expanding.
6. I am enough just as I am.
7. I am flexible and strong.
8. My challenges help me grow.
9. Small actions add up to large change.
10. Today, I choose to acknowledge joy.

INSPIRATION COMES FROM WITHIN YOURSELF. ONE HAS TO BE POSITIVE. WHEN YOU'RE POSITIVE, GOOD THINGS HAPPEN.

—DEEP ROY, ACTOR, PUPPETEER, AND STUNTMAN

WE CAN COMPLAIN BECAUSE ROSE BUSHES HAVE THORNS, OR REJOICE BECAUSE THORNS HAVE ROSES.

—UNKNOWN

SOMETIMES IT TAKES
A HEARTBREAK TO
SHAKE US AWAKE
AND HELP US SEE WE
ARE WORTH SO MUCH
MORE THAN WE'RE
SETTLING FOR.

—MANDY HALE, MOTIVATIONAL SPEAKER

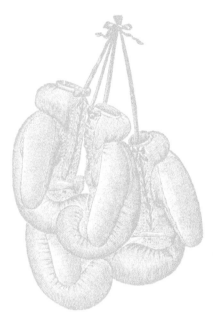

I KNOW WHERE I'M GOING AND I KNOW THE TRUTH, AND I DON'T HAVE TO BE WHAT YOU WANT ME TO BE. I'M FREE TO BE WHAT I WANT.

—MUHAMMAD ALI,
PROFESSIONAL BOXER AND ACTIVIST

WISDOM IS KNOWING I AM NOTHING, LOVE IS KNOWING I AM EVERYTHING, AND BETWEEN THE TWO MY LIFE MOVES.

—SRI NISARGADATTA MAHARAJ,
GURU OF NONDUALISM AND NISARGA YOGA TEACHER

POWER POSITIVITY:
REJECT TOXIC POSITIVITY

Toxic positivity embraces the idea that things are always okay despite things *not* always being okay. It suppresses and invalidates your struggles and emotions. Multiple studies have found that suppressing emotions is correlated with significant health issues, including higher stress responses and even risk for earlier death. Toxic positivity is *not* positive thinking and action. Here are some common examples of toxic positivity messages and ways to reframe them to embrace authentic positive thinking:

※ Only good vibes allowed. → **All types of vibes are valid and welcome.**

※ Just get over it. You survived. Everything is fine. → **It's okay not to feel okay. I can sit with this feeling and let it pass when it's ready.**

※ You should be happy. Things could be worse. → **What I'm feeling is valid. I'm allowed to be unhappy. All my emotions are important.**

IF YOU HEAR A VOICE
WITHIN YOU SAYING,
"YOU ARE NOT A PAINTER,"
THEN BY ALL MEANS
PAINT, BOY, AND THAT
VOICE WILL BE SILENCED,
BUT ONLY BY WORKING.

—VINCENT VAN GOGH,
POST-IMPRESSIONIST PAINTER

I HAVE LEARNED OVER THE YEARS THAT WHEN ONE'S MIND IS MADE UP, THIS DIMINISHES FEAR; KNOWING WHAT MUST BE DONE DOES AWAY WITH FEAR.

—ROSA PARKS, CIVIL RIGHTS ACTIVIST

I HAVE JUST ONE DAY, TODAY, AND I'M GOING TO BE HAPPY IN IT.

—GROUCHO MARX, COMEDIAN AND ACTOR

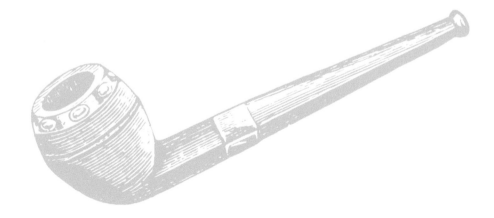

EVERY ACTION YOU TAKE IS A VOTE FOR THE TYPE OF PERSON YOU WISH TO BECOME.

—JAMES CLEAR, AUTHOR AND SPEAKER

Life changes very quickly, in a very positive way, if you let it.

—LINDSEY VONN, ALPINE SKI RACER

POWER POSITIVITY:
EMBRACE CURIOSITY

A great tool for boosting positivity, curiosity is the desire to gain insight into something or learn more about it. Curiosity leads you to seek out new experiences and find out more about yourself. It also helps you gain new understandings of others and the world around you. UC Berkeley's *Greater Good* magazine highlights some of the incredible benefits of being curious: it is associated with higher levels of happiness, it increases levels of achievement, it helps you build more empathy, it strengthens your relationships, and more. Here are some ways to remain curious:

* Be interested in your emotions. What do they feel like? What triggered them? What is the emotion trying to tell you?

* Try something new that interests you. Remain present in this experience. Notice how this experience adds to your understanding of yourself.

* Ask for different perspectives and think about how your biases may limit your perceptions. Remember: Insight is power.

IF THE ESSENTIAL CORE
OF THE PERSON IS DENIED
OR SUPPRESSED, HE
GETS SICK SOMETIMES IN
OBVIOUS WAYS, SOMETIMES
IN SUBTLE WAYS,
SOMETIMES IMMEDIATELY,
SOMETIMES LATER.

—ABRAHAM MASLOW, PSYCHOLOGIST

Turn your wounds into wisdom.

—OPRAH WINFREY,
TALK SHOW HOST, PRODUCER, AUTHOR,
PHILANTHROPIST, AND ENTREPRENEUR

LET US MAKE OUR FUTURE NOW, AND LET US MAKE OUR DREAMS TOMORROW'S REALITY.

—MALALA YOUSAFZAI,
FEMINIST ACTIVIST AND YOUNGEST NOBEL PRIZE LAUREATE

SOME CHANGES LOOK
NEGATIVE ON THE
SURFACE BUT YOU WILL
SOON REALIZE THAT
SPACE IS BEING CREATED
IN YOUR LIFE FOR
SOMETHING NEW
TO EMERGE.

—ECKHART TOLLE, SPIRITUAL TEACHER

TO FULLY RELATE TO ANOTHER,
ONE MUST FIRST RELATE TO
ONESELF. IF WE CANNOT EMBRACE
OUR OWN ALONENESS, WE WILL
SIMPLY USE THE OTHER AS A
SHIELD AGAINST ISOLATION.

—IRVIN D. YALOM, PSYCHIATRIST

POWER POSITIVITY: ENGAGE IN COMPASSIONATE SELF-TALK

The way you talk to yourself is critical in fostering positive thinking. When your inner critic takes the steering wheel, it breeds a whole lot of negativity and shame. Would you talk to a dear friend the way your inner critic talks to you? Then why let it talk to you like that? Challenging these thoughts and talking to yourself in kinder ways can lead to an immediate mood shift in the short term and to positive thinking in the long term. Repeated practice is key! This allows you to build new, positive thinking pathways in your brain. It's like working out a muscle at the gym—it takes practice and repetition to strengthen. Here are some ways to embrace compassionate self-talk:

❋ Forgive yourself for mistakes and reframe them as opportunities to grow.

❋ Take time to identify things you do well and express self-gratitude.

❋ Honor where you are while acknowledging there is always room for positive change.

❋ Recognize how resilient you have been and all that you have overcome in life.

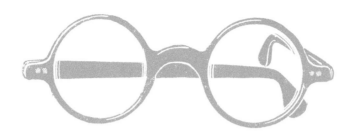

IF WE WANT GREATER CLARITY IN OUR PURPOSE OR DEEPER AND MORE MEANINGFUL SPIRITUAL LIVES, VULNERABILITY IS THE PATH.

—BRENÉ BROWN,
PROFESSOR, AUTHOR, AND VULNERABILITY EXPERT

THEY SAID YOU CAN'T GO TO THE MOON. THEY SAID YOU CAN'T PUT CHEESE INSIDE A PIZZA CRUST, BUT NASA DID IT. THEY HAD TO, BECAUSE THE CHEESE KEPT FLOATING OFF IN SPACE.

—STEPHEN COLBERT,
COMEDIAN AND POLITICAL COMMENTATOR

WE CANNOT BE HAPPY IF WE
EXPECT TO LIVE ALL THE TIME
AT THE HIGHEST PEAK OF
INTENSITY. HAPPINESS IS NOT
A MATTER OF INTENSITY BUT
OF BALANCE AND ORDER AND
RHYTHM AND HARMONY.

—THOMAS MERTON, TRAPPIST MONK

LET HIM WHO WOULD MOVE THE WORLD FIRST MOVE HIMSELF.

—SOCRATES, PHILOSOPHER

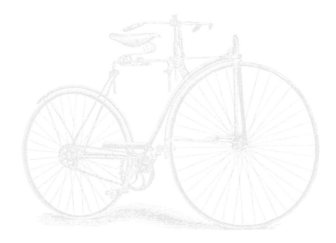

FOR ME, BECOMING ISN'T ABOUT ARRIVING SOMEWHERE OR ACHIEVING A CERTAIN AIM. I SEE IT INSTEAD AS FORWARD MOTION, A MEANS OF EVOLVING, A WAY TO REACH CONTINUOUSLY TOWARD A BETTER SELF. THE JOURNEY DOESN'T END.

—MICHELLE OBAMA,
ATTORNEY, AUTHOR, AND FORMER FIRST
LADY OF THE UNITED STATES

POWER POSITIVITY: SEEK OUT PLEASURE

It may seem obvious, but participating in pleasurable activities is a natural way to embrace positivity in your life. When doing something pleasurable, your brain releases feel-good chemicals such as dopamine, so don't be afraid to feel good. You deserve to enjoy the sweetness in your life! Of course, pleasurable activities may look different to everyone, but here are some general ideas to get you started:

* Cultivate a physical relationship with yourself or with others. Place your hand over your heart or hug a good friend.

* Dress up. Go to dinner in your favorite outfit and flaunt your stuff.

* Throw a party. Make it a themed night while you're at it!

Falling down is a part of life, getting back up is living.

—JOSÉ N. HARRIS, MEMOIRIST

TO BE RENDERED POWERLESS DOES NOT DESTROY YOUR HUMANITY. YOUR RESILIENCE IS YOUR HUMANITY.

—HANNAH GADSBY, COMEDIAN AND ACTOR

I AM THE MASTER OF MY FATE: I AM THE CAPTAIN OF MY SOUL.

—WILLIAM ERNEST HENLEY, AUTHOR

You are enough just as you are.

—MEGHAN MARKLE,
DUCHESS OF SUSSEX AND HUMANITARIAN

FIND THE GOOD. IT'S ALL AROUND YOU. FIND IT, SHOWCASE IT AND YOU'LL START BELIEVING IN IT.

—JESSE OWENS,
FOUR-TIME TRACK AND FIELD OLYMPIC GOLD MEDALIST

POWER POSITIVITY: FOCUS YOUR ATTENTION

When it comes to your well-being, what you pay attention to matters. Your brain naturally has the power to focus on certain stimuli and block out distractions. You can use this to your advantage as a positive thinking skill. Throughout the day, notice where your attention is drawn. Is it drawn to negative thoughts? Irrational thoughts? Flawed assumptions? You may not be seeing the whole picture. Ask yourself if you are disregarding the positive. If so, practicing the following steps will help shift your attention to focus on positivity!

* Notice what is going well in your day.

* Reframe an ill-perceived situation as an opportunity to grow.

* Identify positive actions in which you have engaged.

* Embrace the moments that make you feel good. Try not to minimize them!

BRAVE DOESN'T MEAN YOU'RE NOT SCARED. IT MEANS YOU GO ON EVEN THOUGH YOU'RE SCARED.

—ANGIE THOMAS, AUTHOR

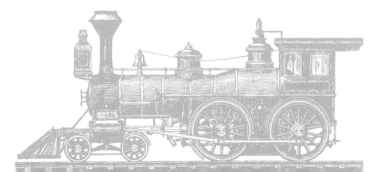

MY LIFE SHOULD BE UNIQUE; IT SHOULD BE AN ALMS, A BATTLE, A CONQUEST, A MEDICINE.

—RALPH WALDO EMERSON,
AUTHOR AND PHILOSOPHER

REGARDLESS OF WHAT YOU WERE TAUGHT TO BELIEVE, THERE NEVER WAS ANYTHING WRONG WITH YOU.

—CHERI HUBER, MEDITATION TEACHER

THROUGH THE DEFINITIONS OF OTHERS, WE CAN NEVER KNOW OUR TRUE POWER AND WHAT EFFECT WE CAN HAVE ON OUR WORLD.

—LAMA TSULTRIM ALLIONE,
FIRST AMERICAN WOMAN ORDAINED
AS A TIBETAN BUDDHIST NUN

THE ONLY WAY TO MAKE SENSE OUT OF CHANGE IS TO PLUNGE INTO IT, MOVE WITH IT, AND JOIN THE DANCE.

—ALAN WATTS, PHILOSOPHER AND BUDDHIST AUTHOR

POWER POSITIVITY:
WRITE IT DOWN!

Writing down your negative thoughts and distressing feelings is a game-changer. The University of Rochester Medical Center notes that journaling about your thoughts and feelings allows you to process them with more clarity by creating insight into your thought patterns, prioritizing your concerns and embracing more positive self-talk. Writing is a distinctive type of thought processing that activates a different area of the brain than speaking does. Writing down your thoughts and emotions helps you let go of them more easily because you are extricating them from yourself. Start small:

* Write down one or two sentences at the end of your day or when you notice negativity pop up in your life.

* As the process becomes more natural, write as much as you need.

* If it's helpful, you could even tear up your writings or throw them away as a form of release. That way, you are creating room for more positivity!

There are always flowers for those who want to see them.

—HENRI MATISSE, PAINTER AND SCULPTOR

THE DESIRE FOR MORE POSITIVE EXPERIENCE IS ITSELF A NEGATIVE EXPERIENCE. AND, PARADOXICALLY, THE ACCEPTANCE OF ONE'S NEGATIVE EXPERIENCE IS ITSELF A POSITIVE EXPERIENCE.

—MARK MANSON, AUTHOR

BE CURIOUS. WELCOME GROUND-LESSNESS. LIGHTEN UP AND RELAX. OFFER CHAOS A CUP OF TEA.

—PEMA CHÖDRÖN,
AMERICAN TIBETAN BUDDHIST AND AUTHOR

WHILE IT IS WISE TO ACCEPT WHAT WE CANNOT CHANGE ABOUT OURSELVES, IT IS ALSO GOOD TO REMEMBER THAT WE ARE NEVER TOO OLD TO REPLACE DISCOURAGEMENT WITH BITS AND PIECES OF CONFIDENCE AND HOPE.

—ELAINE N. ARON,
PSYCHOTHERAPIST AND EXPERT
ON HIGHLY SENSITIVE PEOPLE

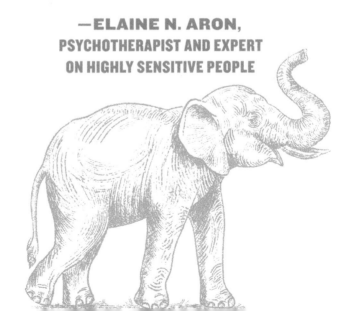

CHANGE YOUR LIFE TODAY. DON'T GAMBLE ON THE FUTURE, ACT NOW, WITHOUT DELAY.

—SIMONE DE BEAUVOIR,
AUTHOR, EXISTENTIALIST PHILOSOPHER, AND FEMINIST

POWER POSITIVITY:
GIVE AND RECEIVE

What you put out into the world and what you are willing to receive can significantly impact your capacity for positivity. The Cleveland Clinic highlights multiple research studies that emphasize the positive effects of giving back, including:

* Greater life satisfaction
* Lower blood pressure
* Decreased stress
* Increased self-esteem
* Increased longevity

Identify an area you are passionate about and positively contribute to it. Volunteering, making financial donations, and helping organize events are only a few of the many ways you can give back.

That said, it is *also* important to allow yourself to receive from others. Do you have a hard time accepting help or compliments from others? Give yourself the gift of receiving. Learning to receive helps strengthen your relationships with others and reduces your stress. If you give *and* receive, you will most certainly find prosperity!

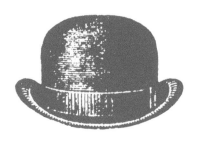

THE GOOD LIFE IS A PROCESS, NOT A STATE OF BEING. IT IS A DIRECTION, NOT A DESTINATION.

—CARL ROGERS,
PSYCHOLOGIST AND FOUNDER OF
HUMANISTIC PSYCHOLOGY

You can, you should, and if you're brave enough to start, you will.

—STEPHEN KING, AUTHOR

WHEREVER YOU ARE, AT ANY MOMENT, TRY AND FIND SOMETHING BEAUTIFUL. A FACE, A LINE OUT OF A POEM, THE CLOUDS OUT OF A WINDOW, SOME GRAFFITI, A WIND FARM. BEAUTY CLEANS THE MIND.

—MATT HAIG, NOVELIST AND JOURNALIST

AS FOR THE FUTURE, IT REMAINS UNWRITTEN. ANYTHING CAN HAPPEN, AND OFTEN WE ARE WRONG.

—TODD KASHDAN, PSYCHOLOGIST

HAPPINESS IS NOT OUT THERE FOR US TO FIND. THE REASON THAT IT'S NOT *OUT THERE* IS THAT IT'S *INSIDE US.*

—SONJA LYUBOMIRSKY, PSYCHOLOGIST

POWER POSITIVITY:
BEND AND BREATHE

A great way to release tension and create more room for positivity is through the incredible outlet of restorative yoga. A powerful somatic exercise, restorative yoga lets you stretch parts of your body to foster deep relaxation mindfully. This practice focuses on being present with your body and your breath as you deepen into certain poses. Appropriate for all types of abilities, this practice is easily modified depending on your needs—you don't have to have any experience in yoga to try it out! This gentle awareness practice has been found to calm the nervous system, reduce stress, and improve overall well-being. The next time you are in need of deep relaxation, search for restorative yoga instructional videos or classes. I recommend practicing with someone who is experienced in this specific type of yoga, as they can help you with modifications for your body's unique needs.

IT'S A FUNNY THING
ABOUT LIFE, ONCE YOU
BEGIN TO TAKE NOTE
OF THE THINGS YOU ARE
GRATEFUL FOR, YOU BEGIN
TO LOSE SIGHT OF THE
THINGS THAT YOU LACK.

—GERMANY KENT, PRINT AND BROADCAST JOURNALIST

INVITING OUR THOUGHTS AND FEELINGS INTO AWARENESS ALLOWS US TO LEARN FROM THEM RATHER THAN BE DRIVEN BY THEM.

—DANIEL J. SIEGEL,
CLINICAL PROFESSOR OF PSYCHIATRY
AND MINDFULNESS EXPERT

Everyone shines, given the right lighting.

—SUSAN CAIN, AUTHOR

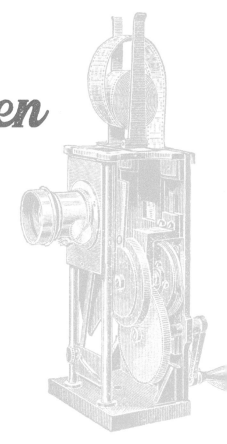

A little nonsense now and then is relished by the wisest men.

—UNKNOWN

WE NEED 4 HUGS
A DAY FOR SURVIVAL.
WE NEED 8 HUGS A DAY
FOR MAINTENANCE.
WE NEED 12 HUGS
A DAY FOR GROWTH.

—VIRGINIA SATIR,
PSYCHOTHERAPIST AND PIONEER OF FAMILY
RECONSTRUCTION THERAPY

POWER POSITIVITY:
RELY ON SELF-COMPASSION

When self-critical thoughts and perfectionist tendencies arise, turn to self-compassion. A powerful positivity tool, self-compassion is the ability to show up for yourself in the moment with tenderness and understanding. Dr. Kristin Neff, a leading researcher on self-compassion, identifies the three common elements of self-compassion as self-kindness, common humanity (all humans suffer, and you are not alone), and mindfulness (being present in the moment).

She also identifies the three obstacles to self-compassion as self-judgment, isolation, and overidentification (making an emotion the main part of your identity or experience). Dr. Neff's research found that self-compassion is connected to reduced self-criticalness, anxiety, and depression and can lead to greater life satisfaction. A 2012 study by Breines and Chien found that self-compassion is correlated with increased resilience and happiness, decreased stress, increased productivity, and motivation for self-improvement. One easy way you can embrace self-compassion is to choose a positive affirmation each morning to motivate you throughout your day.

HAPPINESS, NOT MONEY OR PRESTIGE, SHOULD BE REGARDED AS THE ULTIMATE CURRENCY— THE CURRENCY BY WHICH WE TAKE MEASURE OF OUR LIVES.

—TAL BEN-SHAHAR, POSITIVE PSYCHOLOGY PROFESSOR

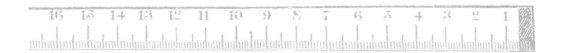

IT'S OKAY TO FEEL TOO MUCH AND KNOW TOO LITTLE.

—GLENNON DOYLE, AUTHOR AND FEMINIST ACTIVIST

IF I WAIT FOR SOMEONE ELSE TO VALIDATE MY EXISTENCE, IT WILL MEAN THAT I'M SHORTCHANGING MYSELF.

—ZANELE MUHOLI, VISUAL ACTIVIST

EVERY PERSON ON
THIS EARTH IS FULL OF
GREAT POSSIBILITIES
THAT CAN BE
REALIZED THROUGH
IMAGINATION, EFFORT,
AND PERSEVERANCE.

—SCOTT BARRY KAUFMAN,
COGNITIVE SCIENTIST, HUMANISTIC
PSYCHOLOGIST, AND AUTHOR

EACH MOMENT OF SELF-HONESTY BUILDS INTIMACY, TRUST, AND COMPASSION. THE MORE YOU LOOK, THE MORE YOU'LL LOVE.

—VIRONIKA TUGALEVA,
POET AND FEMINIST ACTIVIST

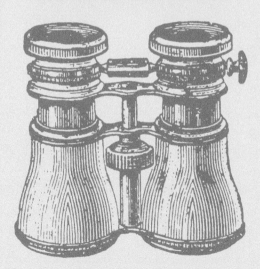

POWER POSITIVITY: GET SILLY

You don't have to be a kid to consciously seek out fun! Keep negativity at bay and further strengthen the positivity pathways in your brain by inviting your inner goofball to come out and play. Dance in the kitchen like no one is watching, sing at the top of your lungs, do improv, watch a silly movie, bake an outrageously decadent dessert, or hang out with your funniest friends! Sometimes engaging in one of these activities is all you need to completely shift your mood from pessimistic to optimistic. When you embrace your specific, authentic interests, you'll find that humor, joy, and positive vibes certainly follow.

A MOMENT OF
SELF-COMPASSION
CAN CHANGE YOUR
ENTIRE DAY. A STRING
OF SUCH MOMENTS
CAN CHANGE THE
COURSE OF YOUR LIFE.

—CHRISTOPHER K. GERMER,
CLINICAL PSYCHOLOGIST AND CO-CREATOR
OF THE MINDFUL SELF-COMPASSION PROGRAM

I WAS BUILT THIS WAY FOR A REASON, SO I'M GOING TO USE IT.

—SIMONE BILES,
MOST DECORATED AMERICAN GYMNAST OF ALL TIME

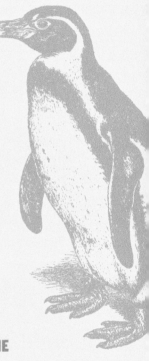

EXTRAORDINARY THINGS ARE ALWAYS HIDING IN PLACES PEOPLE NEVER THINK TO LOOK.

—JODI PICOULT, NOVELIST

HAPPINESS IS NOT DEPENDENT ON
CIRCUMSTANCES BEING EXACTLY
AS WE WANT THEM TO BE, OR ON
OURSELVES BEING EXACTLY AS WE'D
LIKE TO BE. RATHER, HAPPINESS
STEMS FROM LOVING OURSELVES
AND OUR LIVES EXACTLY AS THEY
ARE, KNOWING THAT JOY AND PAIN,
STRENGTH AND WEAKNESS, GLORY
AND FAILURE ARE ALL ESSENTIAL
TO THE FULL HUMAN EXPERIENCE.

—KRISTIN NEFF, PIONEERING SELF-COMPASSION
RESEARCHER, AUTHOR, AND TEACHER

WANTING TO BE SOMEONE
ELSE IS A WASTE OF THE
PERSON YOU ARE. I'D
RATHER BE HATED FOR
WHO I AM THAN LOVED
FOR WHO I AM NOT.

—KURT COBAIN, MUSICIAN

POWER POSITIVITY:
AWAKEN YOUR AWARENESS

Dr. Dan Siegel of the UCLA School of Medicine has conducted in-depth research on the power of mindfulness and how it positively transforms the human brain. In his book *Mindsight*, he explores how nonjudgmental awareness improves the ability to integrate brain connections, experiences, and relationships so that people can create more understanding and meaning in their lives. This integration can lead you to create positive change! But how do you begin to awaken this mindful approach? Take small steps. Try a daily practice of one of these awareness actions:

* When you wake up in the morning, rate how you feel on a scale of 0 to 10.

* Begin to notice self-critical thoughts and label them as your inner critic.

* When you step outside, notice the feeling of the fresh air on your skin.

* When you feel stress, notice where in your body you hold tension.

By becoming more aware in your day-to-day life, you are shifting to a positive mindset!

ALWAYS KEEP YOUR EYES OPEN. KEEP WATCHING. BECAUSE WHATEVER YOU SEE CAN INSPIRE YOU.

—GRACE CODDINGTON,
FORMER CREATIVE DIRECTOR OF *VOGUE* MAGAZINE

Mind is a flexible mirror, adjust it, to see a better world.

—AMIT RAY, AUTHOR AND SPIRITUAL LEADER

AFFIRMATIONS ARE OUR MENTAL VITAMINS, PROVIDING THE SUPPLEMENTARY POSITIVE THOUGHTS WE NEED TO BALANCE THE BARRAGE OF NEGATIVE EVENTS AND THOUGHTS WE EXPERIENCE DAILY.

—TIA WALKER, ENTREPRENEUR AND AUTHOR

WHEN YOU RECOVER OR
DISCOVER SOMETHING
THAT NOURISHES YOUR
SOUL AND BRINGS JOY,
CARE ENOUGH ABOUT
YOURSELF TO MAKE ROOM
FOR IT IN YOUR LIFE.

—JEAN SHINODA BOLEN,
PSYCHIATRIST, JUNGIAN ANALYST, AND AUTHOR

Happiness is the only thing that multiplies when you share it.

—ALBERT SCHWEITZER,
NOBEL PRIZE–WINNING PHILOSOPHER AND MUSICOLOGIST

POWER POSITIVITY:
SHAKE IT OFF

Dr. Peter Levine, a leading trauma psychotherapist, has found that humans can use the same skill animals do of "shaking it off" to let go of challenging emotions. Therefore, you can release distress through literally shaking your body. It may feel silly, but the next time you are feeling pent-up emotion, shake your body. You can do it while standing, sitting, or lying down. Let your body flail around in whatever way it wants to move (without hurting yourself!). It can be fast or slow shakes; do whatever feels comfortable and natural to you. Notice the tension drain from your body. Be aware of any shifts in your mood. If it helps, feel free to put on a song that will help you shake with ease. Shake away to make room for positivity!

BEING DIFFERENT AND THINKING DIFFERENTLY MAKE A PERSON UNFORGETTABLE. HISTORY DOES NOT REMEMBER THE FORGETTABLE. IT HONORS THE UNIQUE MINORITY THE MAJORITY CANNOT FORGET.

—SUZY KASSEM, AUTHOR

YOU ONLY LIVE ONCE, BUT IF YOU DO IT RIGHT, ONCE IS ENOUGH.

—MAE WEST, ACTOR

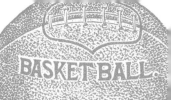

I'VE MISSED MORE THAN 9,000 SHOTS IN MY CAREER. I'VE LOST ALMOST 300 GAMES. TWENTY-SIX TIMES I'VE BEEN TRUSTED TO TAKE THE GAME-WINNING SHOT AND MISSED. I'VE FAILED OVER AND OVER AND OVER AGAIN IN MY LIFE. AND THAT IS WHY I SUCCEED.

—MICHAEL JORDAN, BASKETBALL LEGEND

Here's to us being afraid and doing it anyway.

—GABRIELLE UNION, ACTOR AND ACTIVIST

NOTHING I ACCEPT ABOUT MYSELF CAN BE USED AGAINST ME TO DIMINISH ME.

—AUDRE LORDE,
FEMINIST AUTHOR AND CIVIL RIGHTS ACTIVIST

POWER POSITIVITY: NURTURE YOUR INNER CHILD

Your inner child represents the part of you that is childlike. It's the part of you that feels small when you are in distress. It is also the part of you that has capacity for great wonder and joy. Nurturing your inner child is a positivity practice that allows you to release past toxicity, heal, and take more pleasure in life. Here are three examples of how to nurture your inner child:

❋ If possible, set a picture of yourself as a child as your phone's home screen. Use this as a gentle reminder that there is a part of you that is still vulnerable and in need of your own love.

❋ Write your inner child a letter. Jot down all the positive things you would give yourself that were missing as a child. Affirm that you can give yourself those things now.

❋ Try to experience one new thing each day. Acknowledge your capacity to learn and grow.

FIND OUT WHO YOU ARE AND DO IT ON PURPOSE.

—DOLLY PARTON,
MUSICIAN AND HUMANITARIAN

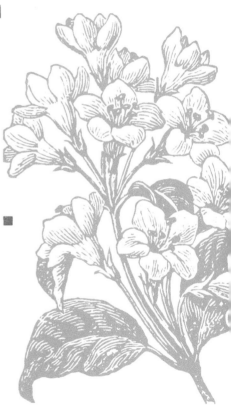

FAIRY TALES ARE
MORE THAN TRUE: NOT
BECAUSE THEY TELL US
THAT DRAGONS EXIST,
BUT BECAUSE THEY
TELL US THAT DRAGONS
CAN BE BEATEN.

—NEIL GAIMAN (PARAPHRASING
G. K. CHESTERTON), AUTHOR

ONE PERSON OF INTEGRITY CAN MAKE A DIFFERENCE.

—ELIE WIESEL, AUTHOR, PROFESSOR, NOBEL PRIZE LAUREATE, AND HOLOCAUST SURVIVOR

WE ARE ALL IN THE GUTTER, BUT SOME OF US ARE LOOKING AT THE STARS.

—OSCAR WILDE, AUTHOR AND PLAYWRIGHT

REMEMBER THIS, WHOEVER YOU ARE, HOWEVER YOU ARE, YOU ARE EQUALLY VALID, EQUALLY JUSTIFIED, AND EQUALLY BEAUTIFUL.

—JUNO DAWSON, ACTOR AND AUTHOR

POWER POSITIVITY:
CHECK IN WITH VITALS

An acronym is a great tool to use for checking in with yourself and moving toward positivity! VITALS is a useful acronym to help you take positive steps toward reaching a goal. Here is what VITALS stands for, as well as how you can engage in each step:

* **V – VALIDATE**: Acknowledge and value your feelings and bring in acceptance. Try not to minimize your experience.

* **I – IMAGINE**: Picture yourself being productive and at peace. Notice how this makes you feel.

* **T – TAKE SMALL STEPS**: Don't overwhelm yourself with too much at once. These small steps add up over time.

* **A – APPLAUD YOURSELF**: Appreciate your efforts and encourage yourself. You've already overcome a lot. You are resilient!

* **L – LIGHTEN THE LOAD**: Identify what you are going to do to decrease negativity. Choose one small action that will mitigate stress and increase contentment.

* **S – SWEETEN THE POT**: Reward yourself with something!

THE POWER OF FINDING BEAUTY IN THE HUMBLEST THINGS MAKES HOME HAPPY AND LIFE LOVELY.

—LOUISA MAY ALCOTT, AUTHOR

DON'T BE AFRAID TO FAIL.
IT'S NOT THE END OF THE
WORLD, AND IN MANY
WAYS, IT'S THE FIRST
STEP TOWARD LEARNING
SOMETHING AND
GETTING BETTER AT IT.

—JON HAMM, ACTOR

HOPE IS IMPORTANT BECAUSE IT CAN MAKE THE PRESENT MOMENT LESS DIFFICULT TO BEAR. IF WE BELIEVE THAT TOMORROW WILL BE BETTER, WE CAN BEAR A HARDSHIP TODAY.

—THICH NHAT HANH,
BUDDHIST MONK AND PEACE ACTIVIST

WINNING DOESN'T ALWAYS MEAN BEING FIRST. WINNING MEANS YOU'RE DOING BETTER THAN YOU'VE DONE BEFORE.

—BONNIE BLAIR, SPEED SKATER

EMOTIONS ARE LIKE
PASSING STORMS, AND
YOU HAVE TO REMIND
YOURSELF THAT IT
WON'T RAIN FOREVER.

—AMY POEHLER, COMEDIAN, DIRECTOR, AND AUTHOR

POWER POSITIVITY:
CARVE OUT "ME" TIME

It's not selfish to make time for yourself. In fact, taking time to yourself can improve relationship satisfaction. University of Michigan studies have found that less time to yourself increases relationship distress. So, I repeat, "me" time is not selfish. Whether it's 5 minutes, 30 minutes, or a whole 24 hours, taking time for yourself is necessary to refuel and help you reach your full potential. Here are some self-care "me" time hacks to embrace:

※ Wake up 15 to 30 minutes early and dedicate that time to whatever lights you up or makes you feel grounded.

※ Make a point of disconnecting from technology and being more present with yourself.

※ Schedule specific days in your calendar for solo time.

※ Ask your family to respect your "me" time.

※ Take a day off. You deserve it!

The next time you guilt yourself into not having "me" time, practice self-compassion and remind yourself that it benefits not only your state of mind and well-being but also others as well. You can't pour from an empty cup!

Embrace the glorious mess that you are.

—ELIZABETH GILBERT, AUTHOR

NO NEED TO HURRY. NO NEED TO SPARKLE. NO NEED TO BE ANYBODY BUT ONESELF.

—VIRGINIA WOOLF, AUTHOR

No one can make you feel inferior without your consent.

—ELEANOR ROOSEVELT,
DIPLOMAT, ACTIVIST, AND LONGEST-SERVING
FIRST LADY OF THE UNITED STATES

FAILURE IS THE CONDIMENT THAT GIVES SUCCESS ITS FLAVOR.

—TRUMAN CAPOTE,
AMERICAN NOVELIST, SCREENWRITER, AND PLAYWRIGHT

No time is wasted time.

—JIM HENSON,
AMERICAN PUPPETEER, ANIMATOR, AND
CREATOR OF THE MUPPETS

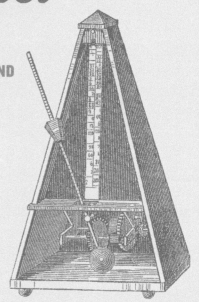

POWER POSITIVITY:
PRIORITIZE PLAY

Playing is an incredible outlet for fostering more positivity in people of all ages. Playing is the act of engaging in an enjoyable recreational activity. Therefore, you are engaging in play when you are doing something fun that doesn't involve practicality or seriousness. Here are some ideas on how you can prioritize play in your life:

* Play with your pet, child, friend, or other loved one.

* Sing in the shower. Belt it out!

* Play a favorite video game.

* Host a board game night with family or friends.

* Sketch, doodle, or color. Get those creative juices flowing!

* Use your environment to spark joy! Build a sandcastle at the beach or a snowman in the snow.

* Throw a themed party for some big laughs. Embrace the extra-silly moments!

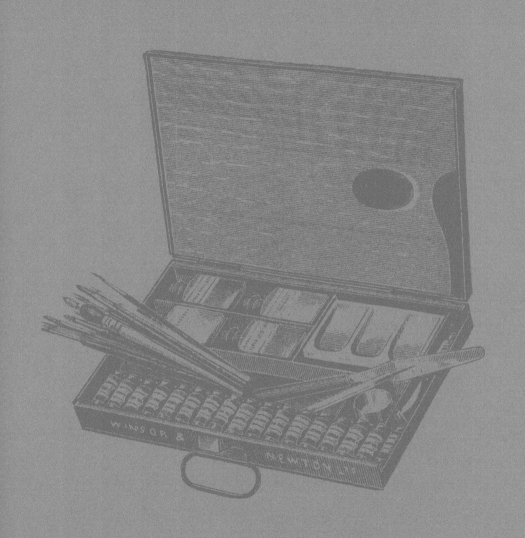

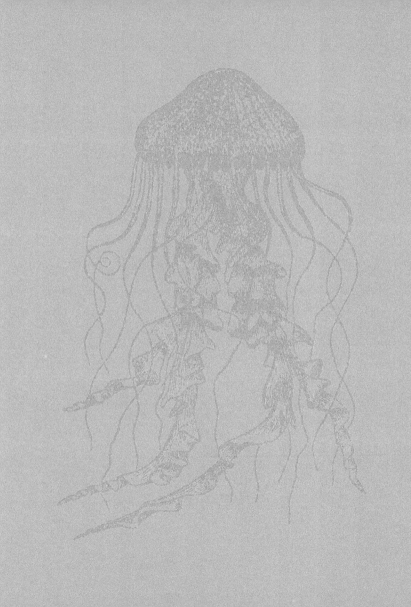

REFERENCES

Bladt, Dorte. "Dr Dan Siegel and the Benefit of Mindfulness."
Switched-On Kids (blog). 2019. Switched-on-Kids.com.au/dr-dan
-siegel-and-the-benefit-of-mindfulness.

Breines, Juliana G., and Serena Chen. "Self-Compassion
Increases Self-Improvement Motivation." *Personality and
Social Psychology Bulletin* 38 no. 9 (May 2012): 1133–1143. DOI:
10.1177/0146167212445599.

Campbell, Emily. "Six Surprising Benefits of Curiosity." Greater
Good Magazine. September 24, 2015. GreaterGood.Berkeley.edu
/article/item/six_surprising_benefits_of_curiosity.

Carter, Sherrie Bourg. "The Tell Tale Signs of Burnout . . . Do
You Have Them?" *Psychology Today*. November 26, 2013.
PsychologyToday.com/us/blog/high-octane-women/201311/the
-tell-tale-signs-burnout-do-you-have-them.

Cleveland Clinic. "Why Giving Is Good for Your Health."
    Health Essentials. October 28, 2020. Health.ClevelandClinic.org
    /why-giving-is-good-for-your-health.

Cohen, Geoffrey L., and David K. Sherman. "The Psychology of
    Change: Self-Affirmation and Social Psychological Inter-
    vention." *Annual Review of Psychology* 65 (2014): 333–371.
    DOI: 10.1146
    /annurev-psych-010213-115137.

Critcher, Clayton R., and David Dunning. "Self-Affirmations
    Provide a Broader Perspective on Self-Threat." *Personality
    and Social Psychology Bulletin* 41, no. 1 (October 2014): 3–18.
    DOI: 10.1177
    /0146167214554956.

Division of Sleep Medicine at Harvard Medical School. "Twelve
    Simple Tips to Improve Your Sleep." Harvard Medical School.
    December 2007. HealthySleep.Med.Harvard.edu/healthy/
    getting/overcoming/tips.

Gender & Sexuality Therapy Center. "How to Nurture and Reparent Your Inner Child." October 25, 2019. GSTherapyCenter.com /blog/2019/10/25/how-to-nurture-and-reparent-your-inner-child.

Hanscom, David. "Affirmations and Neuroplasticity." *Psychology Today*. January 30, 2020. PsychologyToday.com/us/blog/anxiety -another-name-pain/202001/affirmations-and-neuroplasticity.

Happify Daily. "Why 'Me' Time Makes a Huge Difference to Your Happiness." Happify.com. June 2, 2021. Happify.com/hd/why -me-time-is-important-for-happiness-infographic.

Harvard Health Publishing. "Giving Thanks Can Make You Happier." Harvard Medical School. August 14, 2011. Health .Harvard.edu/healthbeat/giving-thanks-can-make-you-happier.

Jabr, Ferris. "Q&A: Why a Rested Brain Is More Creative." *Scientific American*. September 1, 2016. ScientificAmerican .com/article/q-a-why-a-rested-brain-is-more-creative.

Moore, Catherine. "Positive Daily Affirmations: Is There Science Behind It?" PositivePsychology.com. March 16, 2021. PositivePsychology.com/daily-affirmations.

Neff, Kristin. "Definition of Self-Compassion." Self-Compassion.org.
June 2, 2021. Self-Compassion.org/the-three-elements-of-self
-compassion-2.

Oppland, Mike. "8 Ways to Create Flow According to Milay Csikszentmihalyi." PositivePsychology.com. February 15, 2021.
PositivePsychology.com/mihaly-csikszentmihalyi-father-of-flow.

Pacheco, Danielle. "Bedtime Routines for Adults." Sleep
Foundation. January 8, 2021. SleepFoundation.org/sleep
-hygiene/bedtime-routine-for-adults.

Pickhardt, Carl E. "Managing Expectations When Parenting an
Adolescent." *Psychology Today*. April 16, 2018. PsychologyToday
.com/us/blog/surviving-your-childs-adolescence/201804/
managing-expectations-when-parenting-adolescent.

Sherman, David K., Debra P. Bunyan, J. David Creswell, and Lisa
M. Jaremka, "Psychological Vulnerability and Stress: The
Effects of Self-Affirmation on Sympathetic Nervous System
Responses to Naturalistic Stressors." *Health Psychology* 28, no. 5
(September 2009): 554–562. DOI: 10.1037/a0014663.

Soojung-Kim Pang, Alex. "How Resting More Can Boost Your Productivity." Greater Good Magazine. May 11, 2017. GreaterGood .Berkeley.edu/article/item/how_resting_more_can_boost _your_productivity.

UNC Student Affairs. "Check Your V.I.T.A.L.S." Campus Health. June 2, 2021. CampusHealth.UNC.edu/health-topics /academic-success/motivation.

Watson, L. Renee, Marianne Fraser, and Paul Ballas. "Journaling for Mental Health." University of Rochester Medical Center. June 2, 2021. URMC.Rochester.edu/encyclopedia/content. aspx?ContentID=4552&ContentTypeID=1.

Wong, Y. Joel, Jesse Owen, Nicole T. Gabana, Joshua W. Brown, Sydney McInnis, Paul Toth, and Lynn Gilman. "Does Gratitude Writing Improve the Mental Health of Psychotherapy Clients? Evidence from a Randomized Controlled Trial." *Psychotherapy Research* 28, no. 2 (March 2018): 192–202. DOI: 10.1080/10503307 .2016.1169332.

ABOUT THE AUTHOR

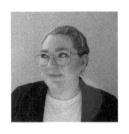

Alexa Brand, MS, LMFT, (she/her), is a psychotherapist and mindfulness mentor who specializes in self-compassion and intersectional approaches to mental health. Alexa has taught graduate-level psychology courses for student therapists and currently works as a family therapist at a teen residential mental health center in Los Angeles, California. In her spare time, Alexa loves watching animated content, drinking tea lattes, and bringing down the racist patriarchy. Contact Alexa at SoulCompassion.com or on Instagram @MindfulFemme.

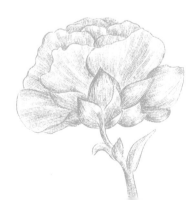